# The Courage to Live

# The Courage to Live

*My Personal Journey with God*
*A Kidney Patient's Story*

Carmen Buelvas Critchlow

Acorn Publishing
A Division of Development Initiatives

362.197
Cri

6/13
gift

© 2001 by Carmen Critchlow
Published by Acorn Publishing
A Division of Development Initiatives
P.O. Box 84
Battle Creek, Michigan 49016-0084
http://www.acornpublishing.com

Printed in the United States of America
First Printing 2001
Second Printing 2002

Cover photo is an adaptation of graphics from arttoday.com.
© 2000-2002 www.arttoday.com

Library of Congress Cataloging-in-Publication Data

Critchlow, Carmen Buelvas, 1957-
  The courage to live : my personal journey with God, a kidney patient's
story / Carmen Buelvas Critchlow.
      p. cm.
  ISBN 0-9710988-3-2 (soft cover)
  1.  Critchlow, Carmen Buelvas, 1957---Health. 2.
Kidneys--Transplantation--Patients--United States--Biography. I.
Title.

  RD575 .C75 2001
  362.1'974610592'092--dc21

                                    2001005600


ISBN 0-9710988-3-2

# Dedication

---

I dedicate this book in loving memory:
To my mother Judith Buelvas,
who taught me to appreciate life,
and to stand strong.
To my father Crisostomo Buelvas,
who taught me courage, strength and loyalty.
To my Aunt Aminta and Uncle Lewis Cobb,
who gave their bodies in death,
so that others may enjoy life.
And to all the donors and their families,
who through organ and tissue donation,
gave unselfishly so they might live on
in all of us, who have accepted
their gift of love and life.

This book was made possible by
the generous support of loving friends and family,
my United Methodist Church family,
the people from Bellevue and surrounding area,
Wal-Mart Store 2080 and Margaret Hart.
Thank you all for your unfailing
support and encouragement.

## ATTENTION READERS

It is the goal of this book to share the author's physical, emotional, and spiritual experiences with End Stage Renal Disease. It should not be interpreted as medical advice, nor as medical opinion about any health condition of individual readers. Neither author, nor publisher, are certified medical professionals. Therefore, this book is offered to the public with the understanding that those responsible for writing, editing, and producing the information within are not engaged in the practice of medicine with the book's contents.

It is not the purpose of this book to present a comprehensive outline of therapies and/or treatments for Renal Disease. Readers are encouraged to read all available material about their own health conditions and to consult with qualified physicians for treatment options.

Every effort has been made to make this book as accurate as possible. However, there may be mistakes in typography or content. Neither author nor publisher shall have liability or responsibility to any person or entity with respect to losses caused, or alleged to be caused, directly or indirectly by the information contained in this book. The intended purpose of the book is to educate and encourage personal reflection.

# CONTENTS

Reflections of a Dialysis Unit Charge Nurse:

The first time I saw Carmen Critchlow, she was sitting in the dialysis chair, blankets covering her from head to toe—and she was very ill. I was afraid for her.

That was six years ago. I've watched Carmen grow during this time. She has had times of illness that we certainly thought would take her from us. I believe it was Carmen's spirit, her faith, her love of family, and the love her family has for her that brought her through those very difficult times.

It has been a privilege to know Carmen and her family. Her dedication to making life better for herself and her peers is amazing. She has turned her personal struggles into victories and shared her experiences with others.

Congratulations, Carmen, on writing your story. May others read about your journey and find the strength and courage to persevere as you have done!

> With kind regards and affection,
> Jeanne VanArman, R.N.

Thoughts from a patient colleague:

The book is excellent and you have covered every detail about being a dialysis patient. I should know, because I have been on dialysis since 1993. I have gone through CAPD, CCPD and now Hemodialysis. I have not had a transplant, but I am still waiting.

Your book made me feel sad, and so very happy, to know that after everything you have gone through, you still have faith—both in your family, and God.

And you're right, God only gives us what we can handle. Sometimes I think I got a double dose. With three teenagers, it's awfully hard. But because of people like you, who have so much strength and faith, I've realized that a bad dialysis day isn't so bad. At least it was another day. Another day on dialysis, but still ANOTHER DAY!

Carmen, my prayers are with you!

Carolene Carter<br>
"Colleague" Patient

Observations of a publisher and friend:

Stories like Carmen's make us both humble and hopeful—humble because few of us have been asked to sustain daily life against such great odds, and hopeful because she inspires those within her reach to grow, no matter the obstacle.

Over many months of working closely with Carmen on her book, I've come to see her as a powerful translator. True, she was born in another culture, to another linguistic tradition, and English has been a learned second language. Even with her physical limitations, she often serves as a translator for the hospital and other community organizations.

In another explicit way, she has learned how to translate into lay terms the complex implications of her disease and the critical need of thousands of patients who are awaiting organ transplants to those of us who might not otherwise understand.

But Carmen is a translator in a much broader human context. Forming local support groups, developing a patient resource library for a dialysis center, supporting other patients who have had or are facing transplants, volunteering to work with the Kidney Foundation, helping others to choose "quality of life" on dialysis, distributing literature about organ donation with the Gift of Life Agency, and helping them translate their material into Spanish—these are only a few examples of how Carmen has *translated* her own illness into advocacy for others.

Although she has cause to be angry, Carmen translates anger into energy. Knowing the underside of pain and weakness, she translates these into strength. Grappling with harsh losses over two decades, she translates disappointments into determination. Her limitations have catapulted her into growth. And what seem like unmerciful hurts, Carmen turns into love. All for the benefit of her family and her community.

Carmen is an ordinary woman, barely five feet tall, who worries about her kids, loves crafts, and teases her husband about the laundry and his collection of reptiles. And her stature in faith, courage, and family love leave me in awe.

My understanding is that the Hebrew meaning of "blessing" translates as "to call forth potential." Carmen has been truly "blessed" and shares that blessing, that calling forth of our own potential, with each of us, who have the privilege to know her.

Doreen Skardarasy
Editor and Friend

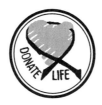

## INTRODUCTION

Before you begin this book, I would like my readers to understand that all patients who have End Stage Renal Disease do not have the mix or the severity of complications I have encountered. This book is the story of my personal experience with how pain and loss have given me a deeper appreciation for my loved ones and a closer relationship with my God. I have not let this illness become a source of weakness, but I have worked hard to let it be an opportunity to grow and learn in Christ. Education, exercise, and encouragement are extremely helpful—not just for us as renal patients, but for everyone. Through these pages I invite you to share in my journey. In your reading, my hope is that this story will somehow translate into an unexpected blessing in your own life.

These pages document my own struggle with a disease I did not choose. Some events may make you sad, or even cry, but please I ask you to not feel sorry for me. Everything that has happened to me has made me a better person.

The following individuals have been my lifeline through the past twenty years. I want to acknowledge them for the strength, faith and nurturing they have shared so unconditionally.

- My Husband, David, who has been with me every step of the way.

- My Children, Peter and Angelina, whose love and patience have grounded me in hope.

- My brother, Ramón, whose gift of unselfish love I will never be able to repay.

- All of my sisters, for their abounding love and generosity, who left their own families to be with me during critical times.

- My mother-in-law, Mary, who has been a mother, a friend and supporter, along with my in-law-family, who have loved me as one of their own.

- Bellevue/Olivet Chapter # 196, Order of Eastern Star, for their wonderful friendship and support.

- My Bellevue Union United Methodist Church family, for their love, encouragement and prayers.

- My Nephrologist and Nurses at Battle Creek Health Systems Dialysis Unit, the Nephrology Center P.C. and Borgess Medical Center, who have been my lifeline and source of education.

- Lifespan Visiting Nurses Services, for their wonderful service in my time of need.

- Wal-Mart Store 2080, which has been a Godsend, providing friendships and supporters to meet me at the front door and beyond.

*"Put all of your trust in the Lord*

*And do not rely on your own understanding.*

*Think of him in all your ways,*

*and he will direct your path."*

—Proverbs 3.5 and 6

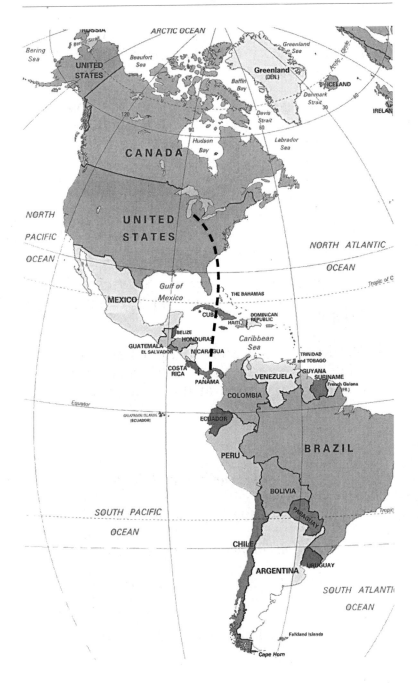

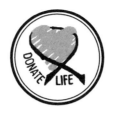

## Chapter 1:   What Is Dialysis?

My name is Carmen Buelvas Critchlow, and I am forty-four years old. I was born in Panamá, a country in Central America. I migrated to the United States in 1971, at the age of thirteen, now thirty years ago. I came to live with my sister in Bellevue, Michigan—leaving my parents, siblings and homeland behind.

It is now December in a new Millennium. Winter is in the air. It's a wonderful season to rejoice and look forward to Christmas and the New Year. Although I am a person on dialysis, today I have so much to be thankful for.

A few years ago television and radio were full of talk about the change of centuries. But my big question was: Will I live to see the new Millennium? I had just survived a horrendous battle with infections, which cost my family and I months after months of hospital time, thousands more dollars in doctor and hospital bills, and countless hours of pain.

There is always one more mountain to climb, but I am a fighter, a long-time survivor. I will wear my climbing shoes until the day I die, and I will find the sun in every day I live.

My dialysis story began in 1981 shortly after the birth of my daughter Angelina. I was diagnosed with kidney disease. My first pregnancy had been easy. Peter was born during the snowstorm of January, 1977. My second pregnancy was neither easy nor enjoyable and it brought complications I never would have anticipated. During those nine months I visited the doctor almost every week.

My due date arrived, but there were no signs of a baby eager to make an appearance. I went to my appointment as usual, and the doctor decided it was best to induce labor. I went to the hospital prepared to give birth to my baby. I knew in my heart that it was a girl. I had the name picked out, and had told my son he was going to have a little sister. Sitting in that hospital bed, I thought maybe I shouldn't have done that, just in case it was a boy.

They gave me the drug to induce labor, but my blood pressure was too high. The doctor felt that it was putting my baby and me in jeopardy. I was told I needed a cesarean. I was afraid for the two of us. I prayed, "Please, let my baby be okay." Two days passed, and still there was no baby. I found myself being wheeled to the operating room.

I had written a letter to my parents back home explaining what was happening. I left an empty space so that my husband David could fill out the name of the baby, in case I was not able to write it later. In surgery the doctors had told me that it was too risky to put me to sleep, that they would numb my abdomen and do the delivery. It sounded simple, until the doctor asked me if they had a choice to save one of us, which one would I choose? What kind of question was that? I chose my baby.

They started to numb the area; they pricked me with needles, and asked me if I felt anything. I said yes. The doctor said he had to start cutting, because my blood pressure was extremely high and the baby was going into convulsions. I could feel them cutting; it felt like a razor. I was holding a stranger's hand, because they wouldn't let my husband come in with me. They told me to scream if I had to, but I said I wouldn't scream, because after this was over I didn't want them talking about me.

I just remember them saying with strained voices, "It's a girl, she's not breathing." The baby started crying, and then they brought her to me. It was my little Angelina. I didn't remember any more until the next day when I woke up in the intensive care unit with toxemia and uremia, which is poison buildup in the blood.

I was discharged seven days later, only to be told my precious baby girl was in serious danger and needed to be hospitalized immediately. She was diagnosed with a thyroid deficiency. I remained at the hospital with her day and night. David came after work to spend the night there with us and in the morning he went to work. My in-laws and my niece, Zari, were taking care of Peter. David and I saw 1981 come in with our little girl at Borgess hospital. We were told our Angelina would be on medication the rest of her life. However, after four years the condition went into remission. Now, at age twenty she remains medication free.

It was at this time I was told I was facing kidney failure and that within six years I would need dialysis, a kidney transplant, or die. Since English was not my native language and I hadn't had much exposure to the medical world, I didn't even know what dialysis was. And there are thousands of people waiting for a kidney transplant. I also learned that the number one killer of kidneys is Hypertension, which is high blood pressure. Diabetes is second. I never had either one. Other than being sick during the pregnancy, I hadn't felt ill. I told myself that I better learn the functions of the kidneys.

Days and then weeks of basic research turned into decades of learning. The kidneys remove extra water and waste products from the body, restore needed chemicals, regulate blood pressure, help with calcium, and vitamin balance. When renal failure begins, the kidneys are not able to clean the waste product or process excess water that collects in the blood and body. When a certain point is reached, kidneys no longer work well enough to maintain the balances for life. This is when dialysis must be initiated to sustain life. I learned that there is no cure for renal failure—only treatments.

When the time came I would have five options.

- Hemodialysis involves a machine that recycles your blood outside of the body through two needles in an access called a fistula, loop graft, or a vascular catheter—usually in the arm or leg. I would do treatments four hours, three times a week for the rest of my life. This treatment can be done in a dialysis center or at home.

- The second form of treatment, CAPD, Continuos Ambulatory Peritoneal Dialysis, involves a catheter being placed in my peritoneum (abdomen) and would enable me to clean my blood and take out the toxins that are killing me. This is done at home.

- The third available treatment, CCAPD, Continuos Cycler Assisted Peritoneal Dialysis, is the same procedure as CAPD, except I would have a machine called a Cycler and would be able to dialyze at home, at night while I slept.

- The fourth treatment option is a transplant, which would mean having a human kidney surgically placed in me from a related living donor or a cadaver.

- The last "option" would be to let nature take its course. Death!

ლ ლ ლ

I was haunted by questions in those early days after my initial diagnosis: Will any of these four treatments give me a normal life? How can I explain this to my children; would they understand? How would my husband carry on without me, if I died? I was terrified, but I knew that I needed to take care of those two beautiful children. My son Peter was only four, and now there was an infant daughter. God would not give me such a wonderful family only to take me away from them and have them grow up without me. Could God be so cruel? I was only twenty-three years old.

I thought of my sister, Judy. She had died on Memorial Day, 1980, in a tragic car accident at the age of thirty-six, leaving four young boys. I had taken care of her children when they needed me. Who would take care of mine? Would I be able to care for my children? Would I be able to be a wife to my husband? What kind of life could we have?

The answers to most of my questions rested on the larger issue of not simply what kidney disease is physically or how dialysis works technically. As with other traumas we all face, it would be a matter of how I would integrate these forces into my life, how I would cope. In those early days, I didn't know. And today, I am still learning.

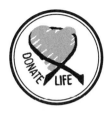

## CHAPTER 2

**CULTURE SHOCK**

I remember how I met David. It was in the seventh grade after my parents had sent me to the United States to live with Judy and her family in Bellevue. I knew that meant a better life for me.

In Panamá, which had been the home of my childhood, there was nothing but poverty and no chance of improvement for me. In a Hispanic household it is not unusual or uncommon for families to help each other in time of need. When I speak of poverty, I am not speaking of lack of money. In my household—and this probably applies to most small Latin village in South or Central America—for Hispanics, the lack of education and self-improvement is poverty. Most small villages in my country only offer a sixth grade education. After graduating from primary school, if a child was lucky enough to have relatives in the city, where more educational alternatives are available, those relatives were expected to take that child and offer a higher education.

When I was a child, I did not know I was poor. We lived like everyone else in our village. Material possessions were not high on our list of priorities. I was living with my Mother's sister, Aminta, and her husband, Lew. My older sister, Tita, had been a member of that household for some time. I was completing seventh grade, when I was given the opportunity by my sister, Judy, and her husband, Martin, to a better education in the United States. In return for that opportunity I was expected—when I was able—to help a relative.

I was not asked if I wanted to go. In my family you obeyed your parents and made them proud by good conduct while away from them. The week before I left my home I said goodbye to my parents and siblings. My mother and father said it was best if they did not come to the airport, because it was too hard for them to see me go.

I was excited by the idea of traveling and I wanted to someday study medicine, so I could come back to my village and help my people. However, I was also full of dread at leaving everyone and everything I loved behind. I know the emotional pain of leaving a parent behind. I could not imagine the pain of a parent in sending a child away.

Once in the United States, I was put right into a local school, even though I didn't know the English language. In my country from the time you begin Kindergarten through the University you wear a uniform, with different colors depending on the school. Males wear slacks, shirt and tie; females wear a knee-length skirt and shirt; and a patch of the school emblem on the left breast pocket for all.

Every Monday morning the staff and the student body congregate in the courtyard for a pledge of alliance and recite the National Anthem and a prayer. Religion is part of our curriculum. In our schools male and female students are forbidden to touch each other. You say *good morning, please, thank you.* You did not speak unless your hand was raised, and you addressed your teachers and each other with respect.

When I arrived in a local school in the United States, I was shocked by students holding each other or kissing in the halls, no National Anthem, no pledge of allegiance, and no prayer. I was the only Hispanic in the entire school. I didn't know if I would ever fit in, or if I even wanted to.

It took me all winter to learn enough English to keep up with the other kids. By the end of high school I was on the honor roll and in the National Honor Society. I had made many friends. I survived those first waves of culture shock and thrived academically and personally.

As a junior in high school I was able to enroll in a course of nurses' training at the vocational center. I earned a certificate for nurses' aid and one for physical therapy. Because I liked to work with the elderly through co-op, I got a job at a nursing home until I graduated.

I started dating David in the tenth grade. In the eleventh grade I returned to Panamá to renew my visa. (A visa is an approval from the government to stay in this country for a period of time.) I was so excited to return home again after four long years. I was also saddened because I was leaving David behind. What if I couldn't come back? I was heart-broken and torn. I wanted to go home to my family, but I didn't want to leave David.

The reunion with my family was wonderful. They had moved to a bigger house much closer to the city and with transportation to the high schools. I saw a closeness in my family I had not recognized a few years earlier. Time and distance had left me feeling like an outsider looking in. I no longer felt part of that intimate family bond they had with one another. I could not help thinking that no education in the world would replace the nurturing and love of a family that had somehow been torn away from me.

After much red tape and government bureaucracy I was granted a visa for another year.

In June of 1976 David and I graduated from high school. I was faced with going home once again. David promised he would come to Panamá.

In August of 1976 David kept that promise and came to Panamá, where we were married. I was surprised by how at ease my family had made David feel. He had learned Spanish and could communicate with all of them. I learned a lesson about family love and loyalty. I learned that no matter how far away from each other we are, or how long that absence endures, the love that binds us will never be broken.

Although David and I were married, even then our lives couldn't begin. David was ready to go home, but my paperwork was not completed. David returned to start college and I was left again to wait for paperwork. For three months I waited, and in the meantime, David called every government official he could pin down until I was finally granted residency in the US.

On Thanksgiving of 1976 I joined my husband David to begin our married life. We had a one-bedroom apartment in Bellevue. Small to most people, for me, it was a castle.

After I returned as a married woman, in the summers I worked for the high school cataloging library books or helping with school programs.

David attended Olivet College. To pay for his education and our household expenses, he worked there part time, cleaning the local doctor's office—and sometimes he refereed ballgames at the school. After our son Peter was born we were informed by our landlord that we had six months to move, because they didn't allow children. Due to the lack of better paying jobs, David joined the Air National Guard.

While he was in boot camp, I went to stay with my sister, Tita, who was now married and living in North Carolina. I was with her for three weeks and then she took me to stay with my Aunt Aminta, for another three weeks. At that time she was living in Florida. It was wonderful to see my Aunt again, because she was like a mother to all of my mother's children. When David finished his training, we were reunited again, a happy young family enjoying our son and our good health.

In December of 1978, we went to Panamá. I wanted my family to meet our son. We spent Christmas with them. It felt glorious to be with all my family under one roof. I had not spent a Christmas with them since I had left what seemed to me was a lifetime ago.

In the Spring of 1979, David found a job with Federal Express, which offered a great health plan and good wages. We didn't know what that health plan would mean to us, and how soon we would need it. David started going to National Guard duty on weekends.

Now we could afford a bigger house. We hoped that my parents would come to live with us, so on a land contract we purchased a house in Battle Creek.

When I informed my parents we had purchased a house big enough for all of us, and I wanted them to come and live with us, they informed me that they didn't want to live in a country where life was expensive. They were too old to change their lifestyle—and besides, all of the family was there. I felt let down. They had sent me away so that I could build a better future, but when I offered them that future, they rejected it. Although disappointed by my parents' decision, we were happy to have a house. It seemed that we would not have to worry about money, but again I was wrong.

In the Fall of that year my sister Yayin's thirteen-year-old daughter, Zari, came to live with us. It was my turn to give her the same opportunity of a better education, as I had been given. Now I was a wife and mother of a child and a teenager, and life was wonderful.

David and I had decided it was time to try for our last baby. Before we were married we had talked about how many babies we would have. I told him I only wanted two children, because I wanted to be able to take care of them so they wouldn't lack for anything. I didn't want more children than we could afford. Deep down I was terrified at the possibility of having to send a child away.

In 1980 we were expecting our second child, and we were all so excited. That excitement was short-lived, though, because early on, I started to be sick with conditions that lasted the entire pregnancy.

Those first few years were filled with the "stuff of life" that occupies all young mothers: teething, diapers, school reports, lunches, transporting kids, and the endless list of keeping a family healthy and happy. What lurked in the backdrop of our lives was the deteriorating condition of my one functioning kidney.

℘  ℘  ℘

In the Summer of 1983, I flew to Panamá, because my father had suffered a cerebral hemorrhage, which left him paralyzed. I could not tell my father about needing a kidney; I had not shared that emotional burden with anyone in Panamá. I felt they were too far, they would only worry. And now I didn't think my father would understand. And I also felt that telling him would only increase his suffering at being unable to do anything about it. I couldn't stand seeing my father suffer. He had lived a full, active life, and now he was in a wheelchair. He had been a strong man. And he had a reservoir of knowledge I always admired. He taught me so much about living in the short time I knew him.

My father was an architect. He built houses. People in our village knew him as *the teacher*, because if they needed something, my father was the one they came to. This included even helping the women of our village with birthing their babies, if a midwife was not available. My father was always there to help someone in need. He built a contraption with drums to bring water into the house. Proudly, we were the only family with indoor water. He also built a huge enclosure to attract mosquitoes and fumigate them to combat yellow fever and malaria.

My father was born in 1905 in Colombia, South America. At the age of twelve he traveled to Panamá and had gotten a job at the Panamá Canal site, distributing water to the

22

workers for five cents a day, so he could help support himself and his mother. His father had died some years earlier. He married my mother late in his life, even though he was twenty-five years her senior. Together they had nine children. Before him, my mother had two. Before my mother, my father had eleven—most of whom I do not know. In Hispanic countries you are born Catholic and large families are not unusual, even today.

ɔ ɔ ɔ

My Father worked hard to provide for us, and with money he got from a disability settlement he purchased a coffee plantation deep in the jungle, away from civilized life. When you live on a farm with animals to take care of and coffee to pick, being *bored* was not in our vocabulary. We were born with a job. My Father's motto was, "If you don't work, you don't eat." We were all happy to work hard, living off the land.

When I was about five years old, everything changed. A poisonous viper bit my father. He cut his toe to bleed out the poison, but it was too late—the poison was already in his blood stream. For days my mother fought her way through the jungle to get him to the nearest city hospital. During those frightening days, my father bled from every pore and crevice in his body. By the time they reached civilization my father had lost consciousness and most of his blood.

The doctors did not want to treat him, because they felt they would be wasting time and medicine on a dying man. My mother had a sister, who was a nurse at that hospital, and she treated him with anti-venom and urged the doctors to give him blood. They reluctantly agreed and gave my father seven pints of blood.

For three months my father remained in a coma. When my father finally regained consciousness, over time he built up enough strength to return home.

He told us an incredible story about approaching a huge wooden door. A man he called St. Peter told him, "Your work on earth is not finished, Crisostomo Buelvas," and he slammed the door. With the slamming of the door, he woke up. He was sure he had gone to heaven.

After that ordeal my father went to the coffee plantation only a few times. However, when he did return, his body would react in the most grotesque ways: his face and body became distorted and he would make the most indescribable movements and sometimes his body would go limp. My mother said he was allergic to the jungle.

At that time we had two homes—one close to the coffee plantation and the other in the nearest village, where my father would spend his time. He realized he could no longer live off the land, and provide a living for his family the way he used to. He had to find another way to offer security to his family.

He found work on a fishing boat, which took him to the ocean—and away from us.

My mother contracted people from our village to help us continue with the work on the farm. But my mother, being a city girl, had no idea about farm work. No matter how hard we worked, we could not make a living off the farm like my father had. My father sent money home every other week to support his family, and my mother took a job taking care of the village.

Before leaving I remember my father telling my brothers to be men, to stand strong, and that men didn't cry. I also remember when my baby sister died, he built her tiny little coffin. And when he buried her, I could see tears in his eyes. My mother was not allowed to go to the cemetery, because she was so distraught. My father told us, he did not want my mother to have the pain of seeing him bury her child. At this time, I could not have loved my father more.

Now this strong man in body and spirit was reduced to living in a wheelchair. Nine months later my invincible father died. I had lost a hero. And someone whose love taught me about strength. I did not know then how much I would need to tap that resource of family stamina, or how soon. Less than two years had passed and my kidney condition had deteriorated significantly.

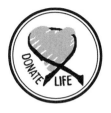

## CHAPTER 3:

**GIFT OF LIFE**

In March of 1984, the time for dialysis had come. I really never felt sick until the last two months or so. I thought I had six years before I had to face this critical stage, but I found myself, a young mother of a seven year old son and a baby only two, en route to the hospital and physical changes that would test us all.

At Borgess Hospital doctors did surgery on my left wrist for an access tube called a *fistula* to do Hemodialysis. After only two days it clotted off. Again I went to Borgess, this time for insertion of a loop graft in my left forearm. When this healed, my treatments would begin. I was feeling tired all the time now, and I was sleeping more and more. I was not sure that I would ever feel normal again. Would this treatment make me feel better? The implications of that question and its answer were profound for not just me, but my family.

In April, 1984, treatment began at Borgess Hospital. I was scared. How will my body react to this? After four hours the first treatment was over and to my surprise I did feel much better. Even though I never got used to dialysis, I adjusted. For eight long months I went to dialysis three days a week for three and a half-hours per treatment.

In the summer of 1984, we took my nieces, Zari and her sister Sanya, to the airport. We could no longer keep them with us. Zari, who had been with us for five years, was of great help to me, taking care of Peter during my pregnancy. And when I couldn't handle it, she also took care of the house. Her sister had come to us less than a year before. But now with me being sick, I just couldn't handle two teenagers and my own small children. With a broken heart I had to call my older sister, Yayin, and informed her I would be sending the girls home. I cried for weeks after they left, because the dream of helping them, in the tradition of our family, had gone with them.

In December, 1984, my brother Ramón, who is a year younger than I, left his wife and children in Panamá and came to be my kidney donor. He was a perfect match, even though no tissue-typing test had been done. In Panamá the doctors would not do a tissue-typing test, so my brother—after discussing it with my mother and siblings, and having faith that he was my match—decided that he was the one to come, and give me the gift of life.

After speaking with the transplant coordinator, and Ramón having passed all of the tests with flying colors, I was told that Medicare would pay for twenty percent of my hospital expenses and all of my donor's expenses. Our insurance would cover eighty percent. Ramón was admitted to the hospital three days before me. I really never had a choice about this transplant. My sister, Tita, had offered to be my donor, but my little brother decided he was giving me one of his kidneys. I was to take it, and that was that. In my family as it always has been, when you were given something—even a kidney—you accepted, were grateful and shut up about it. I silently gave thanks for his love, strength and courage, and also thanked God for him.

December 10, 1984—the day of the scheduled transplant—seemed to come suddenly even after all those months of waiting. My little Angelina would be four the next day. She was at David's brother's house, celebrating her birthday with her cousin, Anna, who was one year and a week older. I prayed that I would not die, not yet. My stomach was in knots, but I tried to relax. Morning came and I was still praying. I made a bargain with God. I asked him to please let me live long enough to see my children graduate from high school. After that He could do anything He wanted with me.

I couldn't explain what happened, but all of a sudden I felt a calm come over me, and deep inside I could hear myself say, "You will not die; the worst that can happen is the kidney will not work, but you will not die." I felt so relieved, like the weight of the world had lifted from me. I saw my brother again before we went into surgery, and I again told him that it was okay if he wanted to change his mind and that I was grateful for him anyway. All he said was "I haven't come this far to turn back now." Again I tried to thank him, and asked David to go with him as long as possible, because my brave little brother didn't speak English and he was in a strange place.

After five hours of surgery, I heard the doctor say, "You are peeing gallons." That sounded great. I saw my son and husband. Still worried, I inquired about my brother and went back to sleep. The nurse came into my room that night to get me up. Moving around, I thought my insides would fall out. The next morning they gave me a chart to keep track of my progress and a list of what medications to take. I was to learn the names of the medications, their side effects, and to learn them by heart before I could go home.

Seven days later I was released with a list of my medications and a Daily Progress Diary. I was told to purchase a thermometer, as I was to record my temperature, weight and blood pressure on a daily basis and bring the progress diary to every doctor's appointment for review. My medications were as follows:

- Cyclosporin: 700 mg taken once a day. An immune suppressant that prevents the body's immune system from attacking a transplanted kidney. It was taken orally mixed with room temperate juice or milk, in a glass cup.
- Prednisone: (Deltasone) 45 mg taken once a day. A steroid hormone, it is an

anti-rejection drug. It helped reduce inflammation and swelling around my new kidney.

- Imuran: 50 mg taken once a day. It is also an anti-rejection drug.
- I N H: 300 mg taken once a day. Isoniazid is a drug to prevent tuberculosis or lung problems due to low resistance in immunity.
- Hydrodiuril: 50 mg taken once a day. It is a water pill to increase urine output.
- Bactrim: 160 mg taken twice a day. To fight infection.
- Tenormin: 50 mg taken once a day. It regulates high blood pressure.
- I also took three Tums with each meal to keep the phosphorus levels down and increase calcium levels.
- A swish and swallow liquid antibiotic was use after each meal and before bed to ease the sores in my mouth.

While taking these medications, I experienced the following side effects: excessive facial hair (I even grew a mustache), tremors, high blood pressure, swollen/bleeding gums, my teeth became sensitive to the cold, headaches, blurred vision, lack of concentration, swelling of the face, increased appetite, (which resulted in weight gain), inability to sleep at night, depression, easy bruising, brittle bones, yellowing of the skin and eyes, convulsions, dizziness and muscle weakness. My hair fell out (however not enough to require a wig), and I had anemia, light-headedness, night sweats and also hallucinations. In the midst of all this, I was terrified that I wouldn't take my medications correctly.

I was not prepared for what I saw when I looked in the mirror. I had gained weight, I had facial hair and my face was full of pimples. I felt like a whale. My body had expanded. I had holes in the roof of my mouth. And even though my kidney was working, I couldn't help but be worried. I was confused and weak. Simple tasks became impossible, and I became paranoid. I was suffering from side effects of the medications, and my blood pressure was way up. Within a few weeks, I experienced a new problem. I was rejecting my new kidney! I understood that there were no guarantees, but how much more of this could I take?

My urethra became clotted and they put a stent in it to help drain into the bladder. It was okay for a couple of weeks, then I was back in the hospital, which was beginning to be my second home.

The first five years after that transplant, I felt like a zombie. I couldn't remember things. I had to stop and try to focus. My brain was in a fog, and I just couldn't concentrate. My attention span was short. I was also sleeping more and more during the day. However, at night I could not sleep, and would be cleaning house most of the night. This transplant was taking a toll on my family and myself. I was always stressed; I couldn't even help my kids get off to school and I was gaining more and more weight. I felt like a real mess. I didn't know what to do. I felt people staring at me and I would hear unkind comments from strangers about my obesity.

ᔐ    ᔐ    ᔐ

In 1986, my mother came to visit. This trip was a real test of faith for my mother. In all the years that my sister lived here and I lived with her, my mother did not visit. She was terrified of air travel, but losing a daughter here six years before, she decided to face that terror and come. When she saw me, she hardly recognized me. She could not believe how much weight I had gained since she had last seen me. She told me that the reason I had facial hair was because I was given a man's kidney. I had to laugh, because these comments are typical with people who do not understand. My mother stayed with us for two months, then left to visit my sisters, Cecilia and Tita, in North Carolina.

ଓ    ଓ    ଓ

In the spring of 1987, I couldn't eat; everything backed up into my throat. I was sent to another specialist. He put a microscopic camera down my throat, and found an ulcer in my esophagus that was probably caused by the prednisone. He advised me to place the prednisone in a gel capsule. To stop the irritation to the esophagus he also added Axid to my medications to heal the ulcer.

Just when I started to feel good again, another infection would start and I was back once again in the hospital. In the meantime our medical bills kept mounting. Medicare had refused to pay for both my brother's expenses and the twenty-percent of mine they had agreed upon. In our attempts to pay the medical bills, other bills suffered. We got behind on our taxes and our house payments. My medications were costing more than a $1,000 a month, not including doctor's visits. The insurance took too long to reimburse us for the medications, so I charged it to our credit cards. We were running out of credit.

Those three years, 1984-1987—undergoing dialysis, the first transplant, the physical and financial burdens of it all—were a testing of faith and family love and loyalty I never could have imagined. I could only offer a quiet prayer of gratitude that God had stayed with us through that test.

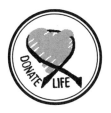

CHAPTER 4:  **LOSS AND FORGIVENESS**

I was in the hospital again. More and more ultra sounds were being done to find out why my kidney was rejecting. In the ultrasound room there was a picture of an ocean scene. It reminded me so much of the oceans along Panamá's coast. I concentrated on the painting and etched it into my mind. From that moment on, whenever I experienced pain or discomfort I would find relief in the image of that painting.

In the summer of 1987, and again in 1988, I had a severe blood infection and for four weeks the Home Health Nurse came to my home twice a day to give me intravenous therapy. I was so grateful for that service, because it meant less time in the hospital.

By the summer of 1989, it appeared that my kidney had completely rejected. I needed a new access for Hemodialysis, because the one I had before the transplant had clotted. For the third time my arm was healing from a graft. While on dialysis the doctor reduced all my transplant medications. I was almost glad this kidney had given up, because for years I had been riding an emotional roller coaster that I just couldn't get off. I was on Hemodialysis for six months when the kidney suddenly started working all on its own, as if it sensed it had a bit more life to give and that I needed that time.

In May of 1990, I traveled to Panamá to be with my mother who was dying. My mother was 68 years old; she suffered complications due to Diabetes. Her organs were failing. Ironically, she needed dialysis to continue life, but she refused the treatments. The doctor assured my family she didn't have much time left, that her body and heart were weak and frail.

As I sat beside my mother, I had to put my thoughts in order. For years I had blamed her for my kidney failure. She was very physical in the discipline of her children. I had experienced that harsh discipline as a child and that could have damaged my kidneys.

I had discussed this with my Nephrologist and he said that there could be several reasons for my kidney failure, including:

① Defective kidneys from birth;

② The fact that I was born with only one kidney; or

③ A blow to the kidneys that caused deterioration over a long period of time.

At that time, he could not determine the actual reason for failure.

As I watched my mother struggle with her own life, I decided to dwell on her strengths and not her weaknesses. Over the three months I stayed with my mother, we discussed my feelings and hers. She apologized for her outbursts of rage and prayed that she did not cause the damage to my kidneys. I loved my mother. And looking back, I am amazed that she survived her lifestyle and all her responsibilities. I knew that for me to survive I must bury my resentment and live with the love that she gave.

In August of 1990, my husband, children, and I returned to the United States. The children had to return to school. I felt sorry to leave, because I knew that, as with my father seven years before, I would not see my mother alive again. She died seven months later of cardiac arrest. I could not return for the funeral due to accumulating bills. For the following two and a half years, I struggled with guilt for not being there, a sense of another loss, and continuing infections and symptoms of rejection.

Deeper than all those symptoms, I felt grateful for the healing and forgiveness that had taken place in my relationship with my mother during those months before her death, and even more grateful for the time I spent with her.

ଔ    ଔ    ଔ

1993 was a horrendous year that would again test not only my faith, but also the faith of my sisters and brothers. In January my Uncle Lew died, after having fought a battle with Emphysema for years. My Aunt Aminta followed him ten months later. She, like my father, had a cerebral hemorrhage. She had been visiting my sister Tita. I got the call; she wanted me to come, because she didn't know what to do. She had also called our sister Cecilia, who was stationed with her husband in Panamá. Tita was fighting her own emotional battle about disconnecting her "Mother" from life support. She wanted me to help her through this hard decision.

My nephew Marty's wife, Barb, took me to North Carolina, because I could not drive by myself. I was experiencing signs of rejection, and I prayed to God, "Please, let my brother's kidney carry me, yet again through another tragic ordeal."

After taking into consideration my Aunt Aminta's wishes, we disconnected her life support. Years before my aunt and I discussed Organ Donation. She told me that she and her husband had talked, and because of me, they had decided to give their bodies to science through Organ Donation. She didn't know what they were able to give, but they at least could donate their bodies to learning about diseases. The ashes of both were sent to my sister Tita six months later.

Our sense of loss was eased by knowing that my uncle had given the gift of sight to a young man. However, we never heard what organs, if any, my aunt donated. My sister Tita, her family, Cecilia, many friends, and I gave both my aunt and uncle a memorial mass. We were tired. So much loss in such a short time.

And the four people who had loved us and cared for us as children were gone. We were adult orphans.

In late December of that same year, my kidney completely rejected all together, and I was back on Hemodialysis. I knew this would eventually happen, but deep inside I felt I had let my brother down. When I talked to him about this, he joked about me not drinking one beer a day like he had recommended before he had given his kidney to me. I couldn't help but cry. He also said that he could give me his other kidney, he would do it gladly. And he hoped I would not ask, because he needed that one.

To this day my little brother, Ramón, has been a powerful living lesson for me in generosity of spirit and gentle humor.

Even though I had other family members ready to donate, I preferred to be put on a transplant list and wait. I didn't want to put another loved one through the pain, and I thought my emotions would not handle another rejection.

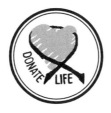

I knew that the waiting period for a kidney is between three and five years. I was surprised at 7:00 a.m. on August of 1994, when I got the call: "We have a kidney for you. Be here within three hours!" My husband was notified at his job in Lansing. Family members were notified, and my mother-in-law, who is also a very good friend and major support for me, came to meet me at the Transplant Center. Within forty-five minutes my son had me at Borgess Hospital in Kalamazoo, Michigan. Upon arrival I was put on dialysis to rid my body of toxins.

As the hour of surgery drew near, my mother-in-law and I prayed for the success of the transplant. I was very nervous, but not afraid, due to my faith in God. I knew my husband David was on his way from work and would be there when I woke up. When I came out of surgery and the anesthesia, the doctor told me it was a good match. I felt really great from the beginning! I went home in two days full of hope for the future. I remained on most of the same medications as before, but only on maintenance doses.

I felt great physically, but the financial burden was becoming a nightmare. Borgess Hospital had been garnishing my husband's wages for the first transplant. It did not matter how much overtime David worked; the more he made, the more they took. We were behind on all our bills. We had collection agents calling day and night. My children were going to school hungry, because we didn't have money for their lunch. And ironically, we didn't qualify for reduced school lunches, because our income was technically too high. I tried to have some kind of food prepared when they came home. My children know that, if we have rice in the house, there is food. We knew though that it was a fine line we were walking.

Before the second transplant I had gotten a

job in a local department store, but after the surgery, they no longer had a place for me. I tried to be positive and find another job.

All of this financial stress was reaching its peak. My husband and I were growing apart. It seemed he was always stressed and upset. We had gotten a notice that if we didn't pay the back taxes, our house would be sold to pay them off. We put off paying other bills to keep up with the taxes.

In the winter of 1993, our furnace had quit and we could not afford to have it repaired, so that winter our house was a freezer. Even though we used the oven, electric blankets, space heaters, and fireplace to keep warm, all we managed to do was raise our electric bill. To complicate matters, that summer our well went out! We paid no bills to accumulate the $3,000 needed to fix the well. We were out of water for three weeks. I had maxed out our credit cards paying for medication. So we could not use them for anything else.

My in-laws did not understand why we were living in these conditions. We never wanted them to know our financial problems. Finally, I broke down and confessed our situation to them. At the time my husband was very angry with me, because he thought I had betrayed him. I think he felt that he had to take care of this problem alone. I also think that he felt helpless, working so hard and not being able to alleviate the huge debt that was strangling our family.

୪  ୪  ୪

Three months after my second transplant in November of 1994, I was hired at the local Wal-Mart store. I felt a tremendous relief at the prospect of being able to help pay the bill. However, by this time the mountain of bills seemed insurmountable.

The day after I was given the new job my mother-in-law and I gathered all of our bills and check stubs and went to seek financial assistance. We went to the Social Security Office, where I had been numerous times before, because they had not paid the original quoted medical payments.

I discovered that some paperwork was missing, omitted or not signed on the original transplant request, causing no payment from Social Security. Thus the 20% of the $60,000 for my surgery and my brother's donation surgery, medications and related medical bills were to be paid by us! Resulting in our present financial crisis.

Our next stop was the Social Services Office. After waiting for hours, we were allowed to see the agent. She looked at my husband's pay stubs and said we didn't qualify for anything. I explained that all our money was going to pay medical bills. She said they looked at the net pay, not take-home pay. If my husband left the residence, I could qualify for food stamps and other services. She also said that we belong to the "Working Poor." Even though everything we made was funneled towards paying bills, because the net income was above poverty level, we didn't qualify for any assistance. In other words, we would be financially better off to sit home and do nothing and let the state take care of us.

The implications of this flew senselessly in the face of our work ethic, all our pride, incentive, and our sense of responsibility in trying to take care of ourselves. I felt so humiliated.

From there we went to Accord, Habitat for Humanity, and the Red Cross. All they could tell me was: "We can't help you." At the United Way I was told that our only chance was to file bankruptcy. I had to admit, at this point bankruptcy sounded like one of our only options. However, we didn't want to hurt Mister T. Davis, from whom we had purchased the house on a land contract. It had been more than six months since we had paid him anything. He had always been wonderful to us. He even reduced our payments.

Finally, we went to the Salvation Army, our last stop and last hope. The waiting area was full of people like me looking for help. On the wall were all kinds of announcements. One said, "We only help with utility bills." I thought I had a chance, since our electric bill was the highest. After my name was called, the lady asked me how many boxes of food I wanted. Not understanding the question, I explained to her that I needed help paying my electric bill. She wrote me a check for the amount of the turn-off notice without question. I mentioned I had brought the bills so she could confirm them. Her kind response was, "If you didn't need help, you would not be here." She was right. I left that office with a portion of my electric bill paid and a large box of food, which only cost $17.00. I returned often for bread, which they give away every afternoon until four.

I went to my dialysis Social Worker and asked for financial help. The Kidney Foundation donated $100 to go towards the furnace. The furnace repairman took one look, fixed a leak, and informed me we needed a new unit. He took the check that the Kidney Foundation had made out to him and never came back. We applied for loans, but since our credit was ruined, no one would lend us money. We worked harder.

My mother-in-law had told my nephew, Tony, about our furnace. One day he showed up with a friend, Raymond, who worked on furnaces. Within two days David and Raymond had the furnace running! For the first time in two winters we had heat. Raymond informed us he would come if we needed further help. He even waited until my first paycheck from Wal-Mart to get paid. Today we are enjoying a wonderful warm home because of Raymond.

In June, 1995, my son Peter graduated from high school, and became a father to my grandson Alexander. I thanked God for the time He was giving me. I was joyous for the good health I was experiencing. And I added a quiet request to let me make it four more years to see my daughter through her graduation.

Early that summer my transplant surgeon informed me that my new kidney could be rejecting. I did not want to believe it, although I was having pain in all of my joints. I began to develop disfiguring calcium deposits on the bones of my extremities. It became difficult to walk and very painful to get dressed. It now took me half an hour to complete what I used to do in five minutes. Even eating became difficult and painful.

Once again my mother-in-law Mary took me to my doctor. She had seen me go through such agony, and if they didn't do something, she was determined to take me to a different doctor. I couldn't even get on the doctor's scales without help. They were appalled at how much I had deteriorated, since they had seen me last.

They sent me to another specialist to test my blood for acid. This test had not been done previously and it showed that my acid levels were extremely high and surgery was required to remove the parathyroid. This is a gland located by the voice box that regulates the amount of calcium the body produces. In End Stage Renal Disease phosphorus binders are required to help rid the body of excess phosphorus, that alters bone reabsortion of calcium, causing deposits of excess calcium in joints and on the top of bone surfaces.

Now, all I could do was go from the bed to the couch. My world was the television set and the couch opposite the big picture window, staring at the road where life and living was happening—and kept on going without me. I lived with the constant fear of a bump or fall that would break a bone. Soon just fixing a lunch became the master job of the day.

My relief came from prayer and mental escape into the picture of the ocean that I had etched into my brain so long ago. Sometimes my husband would tease me saying he had to check on me several times during the night, because I was so deep in concentration, he thought I was dead.

ભ ભ ભ

In September of 1995 I had the parathyroid surgery, and after only weeks I began to feel much better. I could shower, get dressed and I could walk by myself. People who have never struggled with a life threatening illness may not comprehend how even these simple abilities can seem like a gift—a gift of movement, freedom, and independence—a merciful gift.

To even my amazement, within three weeks I returned to work at Wal-Mart. I am very grateful for their concern and willingness to work with individual employees who have health problems. I had been honest with them from the beginning about my kidney failure. And they were willing to hold my job for me, whenever I was able to work.

After the parathyroid surgery, my surgeon informed me that now I needed to eat and drink more dairy products, to build up the calcium that the Parathyroid had been producing. He also prescribed 37 to 40 Tums a day to help supplement that production. It seemed that now my diet consisted of milk, cheese and Tums, and still the calcium was dangerously low. I also was losing weight rapidly, because the Tums were very filling and were replacing other food I would normally eat.

In November of 1995, I woke up in Borgess Hospital. I had a vascular catheter in my neck and the nurse was telling me they did dialysis. My daughter informed me that for days I had been acting child-like and incoherent. I had stopped taking my medicine, so they took me to the hospital. While in route I had a seizure and went into shock.

My body was so depleted of calcium that I had lapsed into hypocalcimia and my kidney had rejected. As the confusion increased, I had forgotten that all the dairy products that I had been consuming were also building up phosphorous and potassium, which was dangerous for a failing kidney.

At that time I also did not know that taking my Tums with any kind of cola, which I was drinking, would reduce the potency of the Tums. And the Cola was also building phosphorous and potassium, both of which were having a negative impact on my body. Therefore, all the Tums I was taking day and night had failed to replenish any calcium.

I was going through only minimal motions of survival each day. I really didn't want to live. What was worse, my husband and children thought I had tried to kill myself. I now know that when the body is depleted of calcium, the mind lapses into mental confusion. Under these conditions a person cannot think straight.

My sisters, Cecilia and Tita, had come to care for me. Cecilia was ready to donate a kidney. We went to the Michigan Transplant Center in Kalamazoo to talk to my transplant surgeon to see if he would do the transplant. He advised me to wait a year, because my bones were still too brittle and my body was too weak to go through another surgery. He also informed me I had spontaneously broken two ribs. Again I would have to return to the Hemodialysis routine. I didn't want to, as this form of treatment is so very exhausting. It drains the life out of me. It makes me weak, tired and helpless. When I get home from dialysis I need to sleep, and for that day I am no good to anyone. When I feel better it's time to go back again, and on and on the vicious cycle goes.

With the sleep that came with dialysis, I would try to forget about what was happening to me. But even my dreams betrayed me.

One dream I remember well was when we—a group of patients—were all in a race, running up a steep mountain. My brother Ramón was running along with me. Whoever reached the top first would win the prize. There were people with guns trying to shoot any one who got close to the top. I was praying that my brother wouldn't reach the top of the mountain, and that I would be shot before I reached it. I didn't want the prize. I just couldn't continue this race.

I really do not know what the prize was, but

I imagine it was the race for life, and our prize would be a kidney. I didn't want it. I just wanted it to be over. My brother was winning. I was being awakened. Yes, even in my dreams the emotional conflict erupted over accepting that gift, so priceless, so fragile, so bound to a life or death game of jeopardy.

I decided to try the Continuous Peritoneal Dialysis. However, the doctor informed me that I couldn't do the Continuous Peritoneal Dialysis, because my calcium levels were still too low and that I could not get calcium through that form of treatment.

From here, it was not only my kidneys that had failed. The walls of my faith started to crumble and I lapsed into periods of self-pity and depression.

My body became ugly to me. I resented others who abused their healthy bodies. I questioned my existence, my sense of being and purpose in life. I no longer believed in my mother's philosophy that "God might tighten the noose around your neck, but he wouldn't choke you." I didn't care if He choked me to death. And for the first time in my life, I prayed for death.

Panamanian people believe that we pay for sins with pain, and those who have fewer sins take on the pain of others, who have more than they can bear. I could hear the voice inside me choking with tears, crying out to God, "For whose sins am I paying?" I had enough. I felt that my body and even God had betrayed me.

For months, the sense of extreme loss continued. I was mourning the life and hopes that had drained out of me. I even discussed death with my daughter and gave her the responsibility of caring for the family upon my death. My mother-in-law, my sister Cecilia, and my loving husband Dave, could no longer reach me to pull me out of this dark hour of despair.

At the point when I felt death was my only relief, my sister Cecilia called and in explicit terms told me to quit feeling sorry for myself and to reflect on the good things in my life— like my husband, my children, and my grandson. It was time for me to move on, live the life that I had and not "die daily" with it.

I took a long look at my self and I did not like what I saw—a weak, helpless, and pathetic human being. I used to be an accepting, sensitive, and caring person. I reflected on my husband, my children, my grandson, my sisters, and how they must see me. I thought of my father and how he fought his way back from death, the strength he had, and what disappointment he would feel, if he saw me giving up on life. I remembered my mother working hard for all of us. They raised no quitter. I had to get my bearings.

As a child in Panamá, I thought I had known poverty. As an adult, I experienced loss of health, the poverty of my body. As a family in a country of wealth, we lived the definition of the "working poor"—a poverty of resources and options. As a woman of faith, and doubt, I now knew the poverty of hope and spirit that may be the most destructive of all.

I was going to fight my way back to life. In my darkness, in my weakness, no one but God could have fueled that decision to remember blessings, to recover hope.

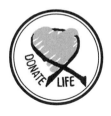

CHAPTER 6:    **THERE IS A GOD**

I was going to learn more about my disease and take charge of it. I would not let
this beat me! I needed to heal not just my physical body, but also my soul. I asked God to for-
give me for doubting Him, and for thinking He
had deserted me. I asked God to help me be a
better Christian, a better wife to David, a better
mother and grandmother. I asked Him to give
me faith, strength and courage to bear the pain
and to be with me through it.

Slowly I began to heal both spiritually and
physically. I made up my mind I would do
everything possible to strengthen my body and
to increased my calcium levels, so that I could
begin the Continuous Peritoneal Dialysis, and

get off Hemodialysis.

In the spring of 1996, during a routine mammogram they found a lump in my right breast and I was facing a biopsy. I was so frightened. I couldn't handle cancer on top of renal failure. It was benign. God had given me a positive sign.

In the summer of 1996, I was severely anemic. Most dialysis patients lose a hormone called Erythropoietin and the bone marrow produces little or no blood. My body was not getting the signal to produce blood. Even though I had been getting epogen shots since my first transplant, my anemia continued to get worse. I was sent to a blood specialist and a bone marrow biopsy was scheduled. This doctor suspected leukemia. It turned out that the Imuran I was taking for anti-rejection all these years was causing my anemia. I discontinued the Imuran, and in less than a month I felt much better and had energy that I hadn't had in a long time. Another positive sign from God.

In the spring of 1997, I was ready to do the Continuous Peritoneal Dialysis. I talked to my managers at Wal-Mart. I gave them a pamphlet explaining the treatment and I explained that now I could only work from 9 a.m. to 3 p.m. Or if I did work in the evenings, I had to be home by 10 p.m., because I had to be on my machine for at least 10 hours during the night. I also told them it was not just the monetary value of the job that was important. I needed to interact with people and to be of value to the world around me. They assured me that I would have a job at Wal-Mart for whatever hours I could give. I thank God for Wal-Mart.

In April of 1997, the Peritoneal Catheter was inserted. During the two-week healing period before the actual peritoneal process began, I decided it was time to help others in Renal Failure. My Social Worker recommended a seminar sponsored by the National Kidney Foundation for Peer Resource Consultants.

Through this training, current dialysis patients, who have made a positive adjustment to kidney failure, become available to support others who are new to dialysis. We don't give advice or try to solve anyone's problems. We are there to listen, and we also share our experiences. I know now that this sharing of experiences not only helps them; it helps me.

For four weeks I did the Continuous Ambulatory Peritoneal Dialysis routine of four exchanges a day. Now I was in control of my own dialysis and I could remain at home to do it. The routine was demanding and required discipline and strict sterility to avoid peritonitis (an infection inside the lining of the abdomen).

I was given the option to go on the night-time cycler, and when I was well instructed and comfortable with the C.C.A.P.D. I returned to work. It was nice to know both processes, because power outages or travel where electrical outlets are not available would necessitate doing manual exchanges. I loved doing this treatment, because I was free from hemodialysis and of the diet and liquid restrictions. With hemodialysis we follow a high protein, low carbohydrate diet with very little potassium and phosphorus, hardly any dairy products, and of course, limited amounts of fluids.

In December of 1997, I felt sick and went to my dialysis unit right away. Sure enough, I had peritonitis. I was sent to Borgess for treatments of the peritonitis, but three days later I was home again. My training nurse at the dialysis unit had taught me how to inject medicine into the fluid bag to treat the infection.

April 1998, my little sister, Maity, came from Panamá to visit. She and her daughter

Maybel stayed with me for three wonderful weeks. We enjoyed ourselves and did a lot of things together; I didn't want them to go. My sister works as a nurse in Panamá, and she was just fascinated with my Peritoneal treatments, because in Panamá Hemodialysis is available, but due to the lack of good transportation C.A.P.D or C.C.A.P.D is not.

In August of 1998, David and I went to Panamá. We had not been to Panamá since my mother's illness eight years earlier. I was excited to see my family again. We sent some of the peritoneal solution ahead by Federal Express and took the rest with us on the airplane. We had no problems with customs, as I had taken a letter from my doctor explaining why I needed the solution. I took David to my birthplace and showed him all of the sites of interest. We had ten of the most enjoyable days that I can remember.

In February of 1999, my daughter had a sports physical and Urine Analysis, which revealed protein in her urine. As loss of protein can be a symptom of kidney failure, I was petrified that she might inherit the problem from me. I wanted her to see a Nephrologist. I had recently been introduced to a new Nephrologist who had been hired by the Battle Creek Health System and was very impressed by his progressive and caring attitude. I asked him to run a twenty-four hour urine test on Angelina. He later assured me that the test results indicated that her condition was not serious and would resolve in time.

Today my daughter is a beautiful, independent and healthy young woman. We have tried to teach her that she can accomplish most anything she sets her mind to achieving. However, some things are predetermined by a Higher Being. She is a very positive person, but like most young people she is still reluctant when it comes to the idea of God's will. I trust her to find her own path to walk with God in this life.

In March of 1999, I felt that I too needed a more understanding and progressive Nephrologist and had all my records transferred to the Nephrologist I had taken my daughter to see.

In May of 1999, I had a second bout of Peritonitis. After five days of treatments against the infection and no signs of healing, my doctor decided that the infection was in the catheter and it had to come out. My world began to fall apart again. Having to go back to hemodialysis again after almost three years of freedom! I was so sick and disillusioned, I even began doubting the new doctor!

I again turned to God for assistance and made up my mind, I was going to get rid of this infection and get back the C.A.P.C. catheter. When I returned home from the hospital, the Home Health Care nurses came to my home twice a day to clean, pack and change the bandages on my abdomen. They were so efficient and caring. They often went beyond just duty. Thank God for nurses.

During this convalescence, the process of aging began to set in. I developed premenopausal symptoms, including ferocious periods. Hemorrhoids that I had from my first childbirth began to bleed and I developed nosebleeds. A trip to a gynecologist and a prescription for hormones eased the menstrual problems and a painful but successful rubber band procedure by a proctologist cured the hemorrhoids. I guess God took care of the nosebleeds. Life was looking good again.

In June, 1999, my Angelina graduated from high school. God had given me life long enough to see both my children graduate. Whatever life remains for me would be of His choosing.

August 12, 1999, David and I celebrated our twenty-third wedding anniversary. The years of pain, poverty and struggle have brought us closer. From lovers to parents, and to best of friends. Through it all, David maintained a sense of humor, always trying to keep me laughing, even when I wanted to cry. David has run the entire race with me. He could have pulled out as he hit many walls, but he kept on running beside me. He has lived our marriage vows: "For better or worse, for richer or poorer, in sickness and in health..." He is truly my Prince Charming!

There are three heroes in the life of Carmen Buelvas Critchlow: my God who saved me, my father who gave me life, and my husband who loves and believes in me.

In late August of 1999, my three sisters, Cecilia from Illinois, Tita from North Carolina, and Yayin from Panamá, decided to come and help me through my healing process. They were afraid that I might have a relapse of depression, which could be fatal. After two weeks Cecilia and Tita returned home to their families and my older sister Yayin remained for six months.

In September of 1999, the second abdominal catheter for C.A.P.D. was inserted.

However, after two days it became infected and was removed. I was informed that due to excessive abdominal scarring I would not be able to return to C.A.P.D. and that I would have to remain on hemodialysis for the rest of my life or receive another transplant.

Again I tapped the resources of my faith in God, a supportive family, a host of friends, a good doctor, caring nurses and my own will to live to take me through the following months.

In September of 1999, I saw my life leaving with the truck full of my C.C.A.P.D. supplies. I no longer needed them. I felt so empty and helpless, I thought I could never again do the wonderful things I did while receiving this form of treatment. I couldn't help but cry. Yayin wanted to know what I was crying about, and I explained my feelings to her. She helped me see that it was only what I perceived as a better treatment that was leaving me, not my life. I still had my life.

My sister Yayin stayed with me through this most difficult time in my life, with her prayers and constant vigil. Although I did not want her to be my nurse when she came, she became just that. At times when I thought I could not go on— or even did not want to—when I thought I wanted to go "through the valley of death" and be done, she was there to hold my hand, to silently sit with me, cry with me, and laugh with me. She is always near me even when we are apart.

At that time I remembered one of my favorite poems and understood a little better what *"Come the Dawn"* meant in my life.

After a while you learn the subtle difference
Between holding a hand and chaining a soul,
And you learn that love doesn't mean leaning,
And company doesn't mean security...
And you begin to accept your defeats,
With your head up and eyes open on today,
Because tomorrow's ground is too uncertain
for plans,
And futures have a way of falling down in
mid-flight.
After a while you'll learn that even sunshine
burns if you get too much.
So you plant your own garden,
And decorate your own soul ...
And you learn that you really can endure...
That you really are strong and you really do
have worth.
And you learn and learn...
With every goodbye, you learn.

—Author Unknown

છ છ છ

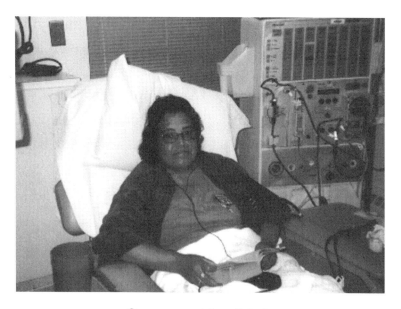

*Carmen receiving dialysis:*
*Battle Creek Health System, Hemodialysis Center*
*Photograph by: Lessie M Terroll, R.N.*

During my time on dialysis, I have time to look around me. I see people from all walks of life. Kidney disease does not discriminate. The majority of patients are elderly, although even young patients frequent our units.

Many dialysis patients have diabetes. This disease affects thousands of people and has a wide range of complications; kidney failure is only one. I understand that diabetics have to take extremely good care of themselves because of poor circulation. One small cut or scrape can take months to heal.

I see these patients fight for life as limbs are taken by infection—surgically removed and discarded as useless objects. I see the struggle and pain these people go through.

As a mother myself, I watch the constant struggle and stamina of the young woman with Lupus, whose only prayer for the day is to get through this four-hour treatment without getting sick to her stomach, so she can go home and take care of her child.

The countless surgical procedures we each have had to keep an active access so that we may get treatment for yet another day. Each of us in that unit forms a bond with the others. Included are not just the doctors, nurses and staff, but everyone from the security guard to the cleaning crew.

Even though we all feel pain, my pain and struggle is altogether different. I only have renal disease. Others have more enemies to overcome.

We are grateful for the people who take care of us, who see us on a daily basis, because for me not so long ago—and for others here— these people may be the only human contact we will have until the next treatment. Healthy people often do not like to be around someone with an illness. They feel uncomfortable or they do not know what to say to us.

Our country is a diverse place with people from all over the earth. Prejudice was not something I thought much about until my transplant. I have rarely been discriminated against for being Hispanic. The only time I have really felt discriminated against was when I became extremely obese, inflated from steroids, which were the drugs I was taking to keep my donated kidney alive. Some think that fat people want to be fat, but many of us do not have a choice.

And now with these patient companions in dialysis—many of whom are isolated because of their grave illnesses—I cannot help but reflect on the odd varieties of discrimination that make people with cancer, severe diabetes, or kidney failure the "outsiders" to others who have the benefit of health. Maybe the challenge to real faith communities is to break through to new understandings of community that do not marginalize those who are "different" or sick. Aren't they sometimes most in need?

My doctor tells me that I have lived the statistics of a dialysis patient. He also said renal patients do not die of kidney failure—and I have to agree—they just die of complications. I see it in front of me. With the many complications this treatment creates, it's another day of life for us.

Death is also a choice we are given, and sometimes it seems to be our only option.

After nearly twenty years of brushing shoulders with these "colleagues" in body and spirit, I can speak for all of us: WE CHOOSE LIFE and everything that comes with it. All of these dialysis patients have become my role models for faith and hope.

છ  છ  છ

During September and October, 1999, I was admitted to the hospital numerous times for changes and infections. During one of these stays I had a very profound religious experience. A Pastor visited me one day and asked if I had asked God for "healing." I explained to him that I had already been granted what I had asked of God and would ask for no more. It was now up to Him to give me what he chose. He explained the Sacrament of the Sick, an anointing or "cleansing with oil."

Later that night I relived that conversation and decided I would put my soul in God's hand, just as I had my body. I asked God to cleanse my soul. Suddenly it was as if God's blanket had been put around me and I was engulfed in peace and warmth. I felt this overwhelming sense of love, joy and a voice telling me that I was cleansed and not to worry, that everything would be all right. I felt such peace and calmness fall over me and was comforted by an intimate presence. That night I slept. In the morning, as I picked up the Bible on the dresser, it opened to a page that read:

> "And as for you, the anointing which you have received from Him abides in you, and you have no need for anyone to teach you; but His anointing teaches you about all things, and it is true and it is not a lie, and just as it has taught you, you abide in Him."

I flipped through the pages again and my eyes fell on this passage:

> "Your sores will be healed and your infections will be cleared away, you will be made clean."

I was speechless. I truly had received a message from God!

That week, when I returned home from the hospital, I contacted the Pastor of the Convis Union Methodist Church, which I had attended.

He came to my home the same afternoon and I asked him about the cleansing with oil. He anointed both my sister Yayin and me. During or after this I didn't feel any different—only happy that my sister had experienced it with me.

In October of 1999, I developed so many infections from the neck catheter that the doctor decided to put a catheter in the left groin. Now I was also suffering from Pericarditis, in infection around the lining of my heart. Fluid began building and I was drowning in my own fluids. I was rushed by helicopter to Borgess Medical Center in Kalamazoo for heart surgery. Several days later I woke up in the Intensive Care Unit. They informed me that I had been on a ventilator due to a collapsed lung and cardiac arrest, and that they had removed the lining around my heart.

By Thanksgiving, 1999, I was home, but not for long. I began to develop fluid again around the Pericardium and was told I would have to be dialyzed six days a week for a month! I could hardly stand my regular routine of four hours a day, three times a week.

Again I asked for God's help, but this time was different. I sensed God's love for me and I was not worried.

Between February through April of 2000, I was in and out of the hospital for repair of multiple graft sites in both arms and legs. They even did a cadaver artery transplant, which is what I am using now. I am grateful for this artery because it is pulsing in my leg, giving me life. Having used all of my arterial sites for graft placement for dialysis, I was informed that a Kidney Transplant was my next resource.

I have been on the Kidney Transplant List since 1995. My sisters and husband have been willing to donate. David completed the tissue testing. This remarkable husband, whose love has sustained me all of these years, was even willing to give part of his body to keep me alive. He was not compatible.

My sister, Tita, has also done the tissue typing. She called me not so long ago and said she had news. I knew right away by the sound of her voice that she was not compatible with me. She said she really wanted to be my donor, but that the test results showed we did not match, and that she was sorry she could not help me. I told her that I was grateful to her for trying and not to worry, because she has helped me in so many other ways.

My sister, Cecilia, is my last chance for a

family match. I have two more sisters and three brothers in Panamá, but they have health problems or crises of their own and are not able to help in this way. I knew that Cecilia would match, because she had done this tissue typing before. Now, she is doing all the physical tests to make sure she is healthy enough to be my donor. I am very reluctant for her to give me a kidney, because the last two years she has not been in the best health. I also know that the doctors would not risk her life, if there were any chance of jeopardizing it. As much as I need a kidney, I am willing to wait in exchange for not causing her pain.

So much has happened in our lives. After everything we have been through, all I have seen through the eyes of a patient, families broken apart because of the burden of an illness they could not cope with, I consider myself lucky to have a family that has stood with me through all the turmoil this illness has brought us.

A man who has been a responsible father and husband, a son and daughter who have learned a lifetime of lessons in their young lives. If I was asked today what would I change, if anything, I would honestly have to say I would not change my family for anything in this world. I did not choose to have renal failure, but without it I don't think I would have learned as much about life and family. Regrets, I have lots, but none that I have not learned from. Today I am still learning.

The only way that I know to show my appreciation to all the wonderful people who have passed through my lifetime is to live the life that I have left to the fullest.

I will take every gift of health that God gives me and open it carefully, savoring every cherished moment. I will take every gift of love given me and wrap myself in its warmth. And I will give thanks to all who have helped me. I have complete faith in my God. I know that I have received a healing. I know now that all healing does not have to be physical. I know I have received a spiritual healing, and that is far greater than a cure. Wholeness is more than health.

God has walked with me along this obstructed road of life. I know when the time comes, He will carry me through the tunnel of death and to the sunlight of eternity. I am not afraid.

From this moment on I will do what I can to help others. I started a support group so that we can help each other live, not just exist, through the years of End Stage Renal Disease. In writing this book I have tried to share how pain and loss can be conquered with love and faith. Two elements we all take for granted.

MAY THE LOVE OF GOD BE WITH EACH OF YOU. LIVE LONG AND PROSPER

*TODAY*

*Today, I will be too calm for worry, too noble for anger,*

*Today, I will believe anything is possible.*

*Today, I will walk through fear without hesitation,*

*Today, I will stand for something,*

*Today, I will make a difference.*

Personal pathways

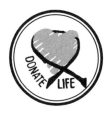

**SOME THOUGHTS ABOUT ORGAN DONATION**

Organ donation is often depicted as a Dracula phenomenon—where life's blood is sucked from one person into another. That is not true or accurate. At the time of death, the body is either buried or cremated and all organs are destroyed. What a waste! *"The gift of life"* for another individual can be given within hours after the donor has been pronounced dead. Organ removal leaves no more disfiguring scarring damage than a surgical procedure.

I know that if I don't get a kidney from a living donor, someone's death could bring me life. I would thank God everyday, and never forget that someone died, and that they live through me.

Living and healthy individuals can also give the "gift of life." That can be given to save a life by a healthy "compatible" individual. Living individuals save thousands of lives every year. Living hair donors make wigs for cancer patients.

Imagine a little girl going to school without embarrassment, because of the donation of your hair to make a wig. Imagine your bone marrow allowing a young mother with Hodgkin's Lymphoma to watch her children grow up. Imagine your pint of blood preventing a teenager from bleeding to death after a car accident. Imagine that your kidney allowed someone like me live the rest of my life without any form of dialysis. We can all live with one kidney.

In the Judeo-Christian tradition, the earliest story of Creation offers food for thought about organ sharing. Genesis 2:21:

> "Then the Lord God caused the man to fall into
> a deep sleep and took one of his ribs and closed
> up the place from which he had removed it."

Think about this: Where would the human race be if God had not transplanted Adam's rib?

Even those who come from other religious or humanistic traditions of belief cannot deny the thousands of lives saved every year worldwide by generous families.

## A CALL FOR GENEROSITY

There was a powerful story a few years ago about a small American child vacationing in Italy with his parents. The child, Nicholas Green, was violently killed in a drive-by shooting by highway robbers. In the middle of their own unthinkable grief, the loving parents shared his organs. Their gift of life went to seven Italian families waiting for transplants.

The human bridges of care and compassion that the Greens built made a tremendous difference. Prior to the tragedy, Italy had been among the lowest ranked donor countries in Europe. In the days after Nicholas' death, the number of people signing donor cards quadrupled in Italy. Last year in that country donors were double what they had been before the tragedy-turned-gift. The world's response to the event is called "the Nicholas Effect." If you would like further information about the continued efforts of this family to promote organ donation, two web sites are valuable resources:

http://nicholaseffect.com/press
http://www.nicholasgreen.org

ଔ  ଔ  ଔ

As much progress has been made, we still have a tremendous amount of work to do to educate the public about the critical needs and shortages.

Transplant and organ donation statistics are changing every day. In my own state of Michigan, patients waiting for transplants as of May, 2001 include 1,718 kidney, 78 heart, 117 lungs, 430 livers, and 136 pancreas.

That's a total of 2,479 persons waiting for the Gift of Life in one state. One hundred and fifty-four patients received an organ transplant year-to-date. Sixty-six patients died waiting for a transplant year-to-date.

In addition, every day, hundreds of people in our state are in need of other tissues such as heart valves, veins, tendons, bone, skin, and corneas in order to survive or maintain their quality of life.

The statistics nationally are even more sobering. The estimated number of patients listed on the National Transplant Waiting List as of May 31, 2002 by organ and overall:

| Organ | Number of Patients |
|---|---|
| Kidney | 52,226 |
| Liver | 17,487 |
| Pancreas | 1,318 |
| Kidney-Pancreas | 2,526 |
| Intestine | 193 |
| Heart | 4,146 |
| Heart-Lung | 210 |
| Lung | 3,777 |
| *Overall | 79,641 |

This data is updated monthly and reported at www.unos.org/Newsroom/critdata_wait.htm.

## MINORITIES AND ORGAN DONATION

Blacks and Hispanics have the highest mortality rate, because of lack of donation in this community.

*Why should minorities be concerned about organ donation? We people of color have the highest mortality rate in the nation. African-Americans, Asian, Pacific Islanders and Hispanics are three times more likely to suffer from End-Stage Renal Disease than Whites. Native Americans are four times as likely than

Whites to suffer from diabetes. We are more likely to suffer from hypertension. Some of these diseases are best treated through transplant; others can only be treated through transplant.

The transplant list for miniorities is long and the donors are few. Just as a family match is better than a non-relative, organ match is best from members of our own race, because we are genetically similar. Certain blood types (O and B) are more common among blacks than among whites. It is more difficult to provide kidney transplant for black patients with type O or B, because more than 80% of kidney donors are white and 12% are black.

Another problem for black renal patients is that of antigen sensitization. Many black patients waiting for a transplant are highly sensitized and it is very difficult to find a compatible kidney for a highly sensitized patient, whether that patient is black or white. High sensitization occurs when blood transfusions or high doses of antibiotics are given to patients on a transplant waiting list.

One clarification may need to be made, however. There are not two waiting lists for whites and minorities. There is one waiting list for all patients. The recent donation of a kidney by a white teacher to her black student highlights that there is compatibility across racial lines. Nonetheless, there are greater needs for organs among the minority populations. So, whatever your racial background, PLEASE DONATE. And, if you are a person of color, PLEASE THINK ABOUT THE GREAT NEED IN OUR COM-MUNITY AND DONATE! All of us will benefit.

Further information about this issue can be found through MOTTEP, the National Minority Organ Tissue Transplant Education Program, founded by Dr. Clive O. Callender, M.D., F.A.C.S. Internet address: www.mottep.org.

* Information about minority organ donation taken from May/June 2000 Community Health Center Management.

## Rumors and Reality: Illegal Organ Sale

Once someone asked me if I had the money, would I buy a kidney? That is a hard question to ask someone if they are waiting for an organ, and even harder for someone whose only option for life is an organ transplant. I know that I would not, but I can only speak for myself. The truth is that sale of organs is illegal in every country of the world, except Iran and China.

The National Kidney Foundation has made a concerted effort to dispel rumors about illegally harvested kidneys in the U. S. Dr. Wendy Brown, Chair of the NKF has said: "There is no evidence that such activity has ever occurred in the United States." The foundation has a legitimate concern that such hoaxes will influence the public's willingness to donate organs, when so many patients are waiting and nine to ten die each day without the needed donation. (www.kidney.org/general/eleckid/myths.cfm)

There are documented cases of organ sales in places like China, where slain prisoners are used as donors and patients from Malaysia and other countries are given a special rate of $10,000 per kidney for transplants in Chinese hospitals. (http://www.observer.co.uk/international/story/0,6903,409218,00.html)

And black market activity, involving the purchase of organs in third world countries like Moldova for patients in Israel have even been subsidized by insurance companies. (*Breaking News*, July 09-31, 2001 http://www.lifeissues.net/related/organ/news/)

However, the sale of body parts remains criminal and unethical in most of the world and to most medical professionals/institutions.

I am a patient who knows well the world of recipients waiting for an organ donation. It seems that the best way to overcome both the pain of the many waiting and the exploitation of the relatively few poor people in desparate countries, who get caught in organ sales, is to foster more legitimate donation through channels of generosity. We cannot do enough to educate the public about the need for organ donation, the facts about how it is done and the life-saving gift it can be to the more than 75,000 people waiting in this country alone.

PLEASE CONSIDER BECOMING AN ORGAN AND TISSUE DONOR.
DON'T FORGET TO TELL YOUR FAMILY OF YOUR DECISION!

• • • • • • • • • • • • • • • • • • • • •

*"Don't take your organs to Heaven.*
*God knows we need them here!"*

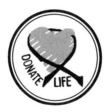

## APPENDIX OF RESOURCES

### GENERAL LIVING DONOR CONTACTS

* To donate Blood call your local American Red Cross. A healthy person can donate every 56 days.

* To donate Bone Marrow call:
  1-800-marrow-2

* To donate Hair call: Locks of Love.
  1-888-896-1588

* Wigs for Kids call: 440-333-4433

* Hair Shed—Natural Woman *A Local MI resource: 68 E. MI Ave., Battle Creek. 616-962-8729. Has a wig bank for hair donation.

* For any Organ Donation or to add your name to the Michigan Donor Registry call: GIFT OF LIFE AGENCY, 1-800-482-4881

* To add your name to your State Registry call your local procurement organization.

## ORGAN PROCUREMENT ORGANIZATIONS BY STATE AND REGION IN THE U.S.*

**Alabama** (1)
Alabama Organ Center
    500 22nd Street South, Suite 102
    Birmingham, AL 35233
    Main Phone: 205-731-9200
    24-hour phone: 800-252-3677
    Web: www.uab.edu/oac/index.htm

**Arizona** (1)
Donor Network of Arizona
    201w.Coolidge
    Phoenix, AZ 85013
    Main phone: 602-222-2200
    24-hour phone: 800-943-6667
    Web: www.donor.network.org/index.html

**Arkansas** (1)
Arkansas Regional Organ Recovery Agency
    1100 N University Ave., Suite 200
    Little Rock. AR 72207-6344
    Main phone: 501-224-2623
    24-hour phone: 501-224-2623
    Web: www.arora.org

    * List developed with appreciated assistance from the Association of Organ Procurement Organizations.

**California** (4)

California Transplant Donor Network
  55 Francisco Street, Suite 510
  San Francisco, CA  94133-2115
  Main phone: 415-637-5888
  24-hour phone: 888-570-9400
  Web: www.ctdn.org

Golden State Donor Services
  1760 Creased Oaks Drive, Suite 160
  Sacramento, CA, 95833-3632
  Main phone: 916-567-1600
  24-hour phone: 800-762-8819
  Web: www.gsds.org

Lifesharing Community Organ Donation
  (Hospital based)
  3665 Ruffin Road, Suite 120
  San Diego CA, 92123-1871
  Main phone: 858-292-8750
  24-hour phone: 888-423-3667

Southern California Organ Procurement Center
  2200 W.3rd Street, Suite400
  Los Angeles, CA  90057
  Main phone: 213-413-6219
  24-hour phone: 800-338-6112

**Colorado** (1)
Donor Alliance
> 3773 Cherry Creek n Drive, Suite 601
> Denver CO, 80209
> Main phone: 303-329-4747
> 24-hour phone: 800-448-4644
> Web: www.donoralliance.org

**Connecticut** (1)
NE Organ Procurement Organization and Tissue Bank
> PO Box 5037
> Hartford CT 06102-5037
> Main phone: 860-545-2256
> 24-hour phone: 800-874-5215
> Web: www.harthosp.org

**Florida** (5)
LifeLink of Florida
> 409 Bayshore Blvd
> Tampa, FL 33606
> Main phone: 813-348-6308
> 24-hour phone: 800-643-6667
> Web: www.lifelinkfound.org

LifeLink of Southwest Florida
> 12655 New Brittany Boulevard, Building 13
> Fort Myers, FL 33907-3631
> Main phone: 941-936-2772
> Web: www.lifelinkfound.org

Organ Procurement Organization at University of Florida
Ayers Medical Plaza North Tower, Suite 570
Gainesville, FL 32601
Main phone: 352-338-7133
24-hour phone: 800-535-4483

Translate
2501 N Orange Avenue, Suite 40
Orlando, FL 32804
Main phone: 407-303-2474
24-hour phone: 800-458-7570
Web: www.TransLife.org

University of Miami Organ Procurement Organization
1150 NW 14th Street, Suite 208
Miami, FL 33136
Main phone: 305-243-7622
24-hour phone: 800-255-4483

**Georgia** (1)
LifeLink of Georgia
3715 Northside Parkway, Suite 300
Atlanta, GA 30327
Main phone: 404-266-8884
24-hour phone: 800-882-7177
Web: www.lifelinkfound.org

**Hawaii** (1)
Organ Donor Center of Hawaii
    900 Fort Street Mall, Suite 1140
    Honolulu, HI 96813
    Main phone: 808-599-7930
    24-hour phone: 808-599-7930

**Illinois** (2)
Chicago Regional Organ and Tissue Bank
    1725 W Harrison Street, Suite 348
    Chicago, IL 61612
    Main phone: 312-243-4011
    24-hour phone: 312-243-4011

Regional Organ Bank of Illinois
    800 S Wells, Suite 190
    Chicago, IL 60607-4529
    Main phone: 312-431-3600
    24-hour phone: 312-431-3600
    Web: www.robi.org

**Indiana** (1)
Indiana Organ Procurement Organization
    429 North Pennsylvania Street, Suite 201
    Indianapolis, IN 46204-1816
    Main phone: 317-685-0389
    24-hour phone: 800-356-7757

**Kansas** (1)
Midwest Transplant Network
   1900 W. 47th Place, Suite 400
   Westwood, KS 66205
   Main phone: 913-262-1668
   24-hour phone: 800-366-6791
   Web: www.,mwob.org

**Kentucky** (1)
Kentucky Organ Donor Affiliates
   106 Broadway
   Louisville, KY 40202
   Main phone: 502-581-9511
   Web: kodaorgan.com

**Louisiana** (1)
Louisiana Organ Procurement Agency
   3501 N. Causeway Boulevard, Suite 940
   Metairie, LA 70002-3626
   Main phone: 504-837-3355
   24-hour phone: 800-833-3666
   Web: www.lopa.org

**Maryland** (1)
Transplant Resource Center of Maryland
   1540 Caton Center Drive, Suite R
   Baltimore, MD 21227
   Main Phone: 410-242-7000
   24-hour phone: 800-932-1133
   Web: mdtransplant.org

## Massachusettes / New England
New England Organ Bank
> Washington St at Newton Comer
> One Gateway Center
> Newton, MA  02458-2803
> Main phone: 617-244-8000
> 24-hour phone: 800-4466362
> Web: neob.org

## Michigan (1)
Gift of Life Agency of Michigan
> 2203 Platt Road
> Ann Arbor, MI  48104
> Main phone: 734-973-1577
> 24-hour phone: 800-482-4881
> Web: tsm-giftoflife.org

## Minnesota / Upper Midwest (1)
LifeSource Upper Midwest Organ Procurement
Organization
> 2550 University Avenue W, Suite 315 South
> St. Paul, MN  55114-1904
> Main phone: 651-603-7800
> 24-hour phone: 800-247-4273
> Web: www.life-source.org

## Mississippi (1)
Mississippi Organ Recovery Agency
> 12 River Bend Place, Suite B
> Jackson, MS  39208

Main Phone: 601-933-1000
24-hour phone: 800-362-6169
Web: www.msora.org

**Missouri** (1)
Mid-America Transplant Services
1139 Olivette Executive Pkwy
St Louis, MO 63132-3205
Main phone: 314-991-1661
24-hour phone: 800-333-6432
Web: www.mts.stl.org

**Nebraska** (1)
Nebraska Organ Retrieval System Inc
5725 F Street
Omaha, NE 68117
Main phone: 402-733-4000
24-hour phone: 800-925-0215

**Nevada** (1)
Nevada Donor Network
4580 S Eastern Avenue, Suite 33
Las Vegas, NV 89119
Main phone: 702-796-9600
24-hour phone: 702-796-9600

**New Jersey** (1)
New Jersey Organ and Tissue Sharing Network
841 Mountain Avenue
Springfield, NJ 07081

Main phone: 973-379-4535
24-hour phone: 800-541-0075
Web: www.sharenj.org

**New Mexico** (1)
New Mexico Donor Program
2715 Broadbent Parkway NE, Suite J
Albuquerque, NM  87107-1609
Main phone: 505-843-7672
24-hour phone: 800-843-7672

**New York** (4)
Center for Donation and Transplant
218 Great Oaks Boulevard
Albany, NY  12203
Main phone: 518-262-5606
24-hour phone: 800-803-6667
Web: www.centerfordonation.com

Finger Lakes Donor Recovery Program
Corporate Woods of Brighton, Bldg. 120, Suite 180
Rochester, NY 14623-1464
Main phone: 716-272-4930
24-hour phone: 800-774-2729

New York Organ Donor Network
475 Riverside Driv, Suite 1244
New York, NY  10115-1244
Web: www.nyodn.org

Upstate New York Transplant Services Inc
  165 Genesee Street, Suite 102
  Buffalo, NY  14203
  Main phone: 715-853-6667
  24-hour phone: 800-227-4771 Web: www.unyts.org

**North Carolina** (2)
Carolina Donor Services
  702 Johns Hopkins Drive
  Greenville, NC  27834
  Main phone: 252-757-0090
  24-hour phone: 252-752-5480
  Web: www.copanc.org

Lifeshare of the Carolinas
  (Hospital-based)
  PO Box 32861
  Charlotte, NC  28232-2861
  Main phone: 704-548-6850
  24-hour phone: 800-932-4483

**Ohio** (4)
Life Connection of Ohio
  1545 Holland Road, Suite C
  Maumee, OH  43537-1694
  Main phone: 419-893-4891
  24-hour phone: 800-535-9206 Web:
  www.mco.edu/hosp/lifecom

LifeBanc

    20600 Chagrin Boulevard, Suite 350

    Cleveland, OH 44122-5343

    Main phone: 216-752-5433

    24-hour phone: 800-558-5433

    Web: www.lifebanc.org

Lifeline of Ohio

    770 Kinnear Road, Suite 200

    Columbus, OH 43212

    Main phone: 614-291-5667

    24-hour phone: 800-525-5667

    Web: www.lifelineofohio,org

Ohio Valley LifeCenter

    2925 Vernon Place, Suite 300

    Cincinnati, OH 45219-2430

    Main phone: 513-558-5555

    24-hour phone: 513-558-5000

    Web: www.lifecnt.org

**Oklahoma** (2)

Hillcrest Medical Center OPO

    (Hospital-based)

    1120 S Utica Avenue

    Tulsa, OK 74104

    Main phone: 918-579-1000

    24-hour phone: 918-579-1000

Oklahoma Organ Sharing Network
   5801 N Broadway, Suite 100
   Oklahoma City, OK  73118-7489
   Main phone: 405-840-5551
   24-hour phone: 800-241-4483
   Web: www.oosn.com

**Oregon / Pacific Northwest**
Pacific Northwest Transplant Bank
   2611 S. W. Third Avenue, Suite 320
   Portland, OR  97201
   Main phone: 503-494-5560
   24-hour phone: 800-344-8916

**Pennsylvania** (2)
Center for Organ Recovery and Education
   204 Sigma Drive
   RIDC Park
   Pittsburgh, PA 15238-2825
   Main phone: 412-963-3550
   24-hour phone: 800-366-6777
   Web: www.core.org

Gift of Life Donor Program
   2000 Hamilton Street
   Rodin Pl. Suite 201
   Philadelphia, PA  19130-3813
   Main phone: 215-557-8090
   24-hour phone: 800-543-6391
   Web: www.donors1.org

**Puerto Rico** (1)
Life Link of Puerto Rico
Campag Centre
Suite 402
Guaynabo PR  00968-1702
Main phone: 787-277-0900
24-hour phone: 800-558-0907 Web: lifelink@prtc.net

**South Carolina** (1)
South Carolina Organ Procurement Agency
1064 Gardner Road
Suite 105
Charleston, SC  29407
Main phone: 843-763-7755
24-hour phone: 800-462-0755
Web: www.scopa.org

**Tennessee / Mid-South** (2)
Mid-South Transplant Foundation
910 Madison Avenue
10th Floor
Memphis, TN  38103
Main phone: 901-328-4438
24-hour phone: 901-366-6775
Web: www.midsouthtransplant.org

Tennessee Donor Services
1714 Hayes Street
Nashville, TN  37203
Main phone: 615-234-5251
24-hour phone: 615-327-2247 Web:
www.kormet.org/donor

**Texas** (1)
LifeGift Organ Donation Center
    5615 Kirby Drive, Suite 900
    Houston, TX 77005-2405
    Main phone: 713-523-4438
    24-hour phone: 713-737-8111
    Web: www.lifegift.org

**Utah** (1)
Intermountain Organ Recovery System
    230 S 500 East, Suite290
    Salt Lake City, UT 84102
    Main phone: 801-521-1755
    24-hour phone: 800-833-6667
    Web: www.iors.com

**Virginia** (3)
LifeNet
    5809 Ward Court
    Virginia Beach, VA 23455-3312
    Main phone: 757-464-4761
    24-hour: 800-847-7831
    Web: www.life-net.org

Virginias Organ Procurement Agency
    8154 Forest Hill Avenue, Suite 4
    Richmond, VA 23235
    Main phone: 804-330-0800
    24-hour phone: 800-233-8672

Washington Regional Transplant Consortium
    8110 Gatehouse Road, Suite 101 West
    Falls Church, VA  22042
    Main phone: 703-641-0100
    24-phone: 703-641-0100 Web: www.wrtc.org

**Washington** (1)
Lifecenter Northwest Donor Network
    2553 76th Avenue SE
    Mercer Island, WA  98040
    Main phone: 206-230-5767
    24-hour phone: 888-543-3287
    Web: www.icnw.org/donation fs.html

**Wisconsin** (2)
Organ Procurement Organization at Univ. of WI
    600 Highland Avenue
    Madison, WI  53792
    Main phone: 608-263-1341
    24-hour phone: 608-262-0143
    Web: www.surgery.wisc.edu

Wisconsin Donor Network
    (Hospital-based)
    9200 W Wisconsin Avenue
    Milwaukee, WI  53226
    Main phone: 414-259-2024
    24-hour phone: 800-432-5405

## ABOUT TRAVEL

### A. EMERGENCY TRAVEL PACK FOR HEMODIALYSIS:

◆ DAILY check your access site for a pulse, whether away or at home.

◆ NEVER hang a purse or bag from your shoulder of your access arm.

◆ NEVER push or hold anything with your access leg.

◆ ALWAYS check for signs of infection:
   1. Warm access
   2. Red access
   3. Swollen access, legs or feet
   4. Fever
   5. Chills

◆ ALWAYS have with you:
   1. Salt
   2. Gauze, sponges
   3. Tape
   4. List of all your medications, how much you take, and what doctor prescribed it
   5. List of your Nephrologist and emergency contact numbers.

◆ ALWAYS (if traveling by air or train) carry medications with you, take extra in case of you don't get home as expected.

- If your Social Worker made arrangements for you to be dialyzed in a different unit, ALWAYS call ahead yourself to ask questions of what is acceptable in that unit. (visitors, food, drink, blanket).

- And most important, know your **Arterial Site** from your **Venous Site**, and know if it is shallow or deep, since all sites are not the same.

## B. EMERGENCY TRAVEL PACK FOR CAPD:

- I V pole

- Betadine

- Blood pressure cuff

- Thermometer

- Solution and tubing (take enough solution and tubing for a couple of extra days in case you are delayed)

- Masks

- Paper towels or moist toilettes

- Heating pad

- Don't forget to take an empty solution bag for your waste

- Name of medications and Doctor who prescribed it

- Name and number of emergency contact person.

## C. EMERGENCY TRAVEL PACK FOR CCAPD:

◆ Same as above except omit the I V pole and take your Clycler.

◆ Don't forget to take a universal electrical plug converter in case you can't find a 3-prong outlet.

◆ Also take with you a list of CCAPD units available in that area in case of emergency

◆ ALWAYS have with you a universal catheter adapter, because if you need emergency supplies from a different unit the tubing may not be the same; you will need to adapt it to yours.

◆ If you don't know what a universal adapter is, ask your nurse.

◆ Away and at home ALWAYS check for signs of infection.

◆ Check site for redness or soreness.
1. Cloudy outflow
2. Abdominal cramps
3. Nausea-vomiting
4. Fever-chills
5. Swollen abdomen, legs or feet

◆ NEVER NEVER FORGET YOUR STERILE TECHNIQUE:
1. Secure your treatment area before you start your treatment.
2. Always: wash & dry hands, wear your mask, take your time.

3. No pets in the room.

4. Daily showers (Important to remember: don't dry with the "community" towel or use bar soap. Use body wash instead, as bar soap harbors bacteria.)

5. Close all potential drafts.

## ABOUT MEDICATION:

• Always take your medications as prescribed.

• Know what new medications are for and what the side effects are for each medication you take.

• Don't take blood pressure pill, water or heart pill, together. They will all lower your blood pressure.

• Take your iron pills two hours before or after your Phoslo; otherwise, they will counter-react and kill the potency of each other.

• Remember: any kind of Cola will raise your potassium and phosphorous levels, and also will diminish the potency of the Phoslo.

• Ask your doctor to review periodically with you what foods or liquids might conflict with your treatment and/or your medications. Each time your medication changes, ask the question again. There have been times when my health was placed at grave risk due to foods in conflict with my medication or treatment. We can all say: "They—the medical professionals—should have told me." But it is safest for us to always ask the question, before it is too late.

## ABOUT PAIN AND COPING WITH PHYSICAL LIMITATIONS:

♦ I have learned how to control some pain with a deep concentration of a picture or a childhood memory. In my mind's eye I have etched happy memories of my childhood in my village or by the ocean. Another image I have used successfully is related to stories from my own religious up-bringing. Although I've never been to the Holy Land, I have seen pictures or television scenes of Jesus walking into the River Jordan, or in the multitude with hordes of people asking to be healed. I lay really still, and concentrate to a point of a trance. I take myself there and almost walk among them and touch His robe. And for a while I feel no pain, or it is diminished. I learned this technique from Doris, a lay person in my church. She has been an inspiration for my spiritual health.

This is a learned skill anyone can master. It only takes practice concentrating and is well worth the effort.

First you need to concentrate on a picture or a happy memory and place it in your mind. You need to teach yourself to relax your entire body before you can relax your mind. Lay still, take deep breaths through your nose, count to 10 very slowly, exhale through your mouth, again very slowly, repeating the process until you feel the weight on your body and mind lighten. Place the picture in your mind and go there. This is what I do; it may not necessarily work for you.

Each of us has to find our own way to relax.

*MindBody Cancer Wellness*, written by Dr. Morry Edwards, offers a wide range of techniques he has successfully taught patients with serious illnesses for more than 20 years. ISBN 0-9710988-0-8. (Available through www.acornpublishing.com)

♦ Remember the things that give you life and energy.

During periods when I am not terribly sick, I like to do crafts. They keep me busy and take my mind off of myself. My family says that if I have plaster, wood, paint, and cement, I am happy. They are right. I like to create things, rather than dwell on what I can do nothing about.

What I am trying to say is: let yourself feel and act with purpose. If you had a job before this disease and now you can't work, find a hobby. Do volunteer work. Volunteering is a great way to keep your mind off your illness and help others. The key is to keep busy with things you want to do.

Music is also a wonderful therapeutic activity. I don't know where I'd be without my Spanish music. When I am depressed, I just turn my music full blast. Who can be low when Mambo, Cumbia or Zamba music is playing?

What is it for you? Arts and crafts, reading, sewing, houseplants, flowers in the garden, Bonsai trees, antique toys, National Geographic specials, movies, learning a new language, music, collecting stones, volunteering? Whatever it is that lends joy, comfort, or a sense of ordinary feel-good daily life—tap those things, enjoy them, share them with people who love you. These will help keep you, and

your loved ones, mentally, emotionally and psycho-
logically healthy and positive. And remember that
your spouse or most immediate family members
have this same need for tapping life resources. My
husband's growing collection of reptiles and trop-
ical plants give him life and an outlet, when illness
might be overwhelming.

◆ Don't forget to laugh. Humor might be one of the
most important healing forces that is often neglected,
when we are physically fighting for a quality of life
that will defy an illness like Renal Failure. This
might be a great time to reflect on who and what
makes you laugh, what lifts the heaviness of illness
even for moments at a time. One thing that has
always helped our family is my husband's doing
impressions of Mr. Bean, the famous British come-
dian. If it's Mr. Bean, then have "him" to dinner
through a video. If it's Laurel and Hardy, find a col-
lector's edition at the local library. If it's what children say, put your hands on an old Art Linklighter
book or visit a neighbor with small children.

◆ Most Dialysis Units have information on how to
cope with Kidney disease. I've attended the R.I.S.E
Rehabilitation, Information, Support and Empow-
erment. It is a four-day seminar sponsored by the
National Kidney Foundation. It teaches you all you
need to know about having quality of life living
with Renal Failure. They will give you a list of
magazines you can subscribe to and some are free.
For a R.I.S.E seminar nearest you, call your local
Kidney Foundation. This Foundation also has
books on Kidney Disease and Dialysis, Kidney
Dialysis and the family. They also have cookbooks

for the dialysis patient. (This you may have to purchase.)

♦ In the final analysis, it is important to keep in mind that none of us are invincible. As *Common Concerns,* the newsletter from the Kidney Foundation, points out, depression is very common among people who are on dialysis. If you are experiencing something that is more than a few days of "the blues," you may have something that more closely resembles clinical depression. Seek out resources that might help. Ask your doctor about ways to cope with your depression. Ask, and be open to speaking with a counselor. Research at the library or on the internet. Don't let depression zap you of more life. There are ways to cope with it, even for those of us with Kidney Disease.

Some useful resources include:

www.depression.about.com

www.nimh.nih.gov

www.intimacyanddepression.com

www.youngadultsdepression.homestead.com/
depression100.html

## SPIRITUAL RESOURCES

♦ The BIBLE. In this book you will find the road to happiness and contentment. You will find out that happiness does not come from other people but from within yourself. No one can make you happy, you need to look deep inside you to find your own happiness. God can give you happiness. The Joy in the Lord can bring you strength. In this book you will find that if you practice love and respect for others everyday, you will be fulfilled.

◆ *GOD CALLING. A Devotional Diary* written by two women who elected to remain anonymous. Edited by A.J. Russell.

A Teacher and a role model, on my high school graduation gave it to me. This daily devotional has helped tremendously in calming my fears on a day-to-day basis. When I feel depressed of unsure of myself, I look to this book for reassurance and I find it. Today it reads:

### God-Inspired

*You have entered now upon a mountain climb. Steep steps lead upward, but your power to help others will be truly marvelous.*

*Not alone will you arise. All towards whom you now send loving, pitying thoughts will be helped upward by you.*

*Looking to Me all your thoughts are God-inspired. Act on them and you will be led on. They are not your own impulses but the movement of My Spirit and, obeyed, will bring the answer to your prayers. Love and Trust. Let no unkind thoughts of any dwell in your hearts, then I can act with all My Spirit-Power, with nothing to hinder.*

◆ Joyce Meyer is a minister, who has produced wonderful inspirational books and tapes. You can find them at most Christian bookstores or at her website:

www.joycemeyer.org   A few that I've especially liked have been: *Improving Relationships* (4 tape series), *How to Handle and Deal with Anger* (5 tape series), and *Reduce Me to Love. Unlocking the Secret to Lasting Joy.*

♦ And, ALWAYS RELY ON THE LOVE OF GOD. For me it is OUR FATHER, JESUS CHRIST HIS SON WHO IS OUR SOURCE OF STRENGH AND COURAGE, AND THE POWER OF GOD THOUGH THE HOLY SPIRIT. I believe that IF YOU ASK, OUR GOD WILL NEVER LEAVE YOU.

♦ If your faith rests in another religious tradition, then let it be strengthened by forms of prayer that you give you comfort.

♦ And if you have never prayed, never been exposed to traditional paths that invited you to grow spiritually, then in your solitude ask the Spirit who dwells within you to be present. Maybe the words, "The Kingdom of God is within you" were meant for all of us, regardless of our theology.

♦ There are literally thousands of resources in the form of books, audiotapes, videos, individuals and organizations dedicated to helping us cope better and find the spiritual meaning we need, even, maybe especially, when we are dealing with an illness like Kidney Disease. Don't starve yourself spiritually, when there is a banquet of resources within reach in the community, bookstores, libraries, and the internet.

## ABOUT YOU AND COMMUNITY

I have tried to give you as much information as I could in this book. Although my physical conditions have been extreme, please know that even I can confirm that THERE IS LIFE AFTER DIALYSIS. Living with dialysis or the complications from transplants is not easy, but you CAN do it.

◆ Rely on the loving support of family and friends. Keep lines of communication open with your personal lifelines. Remember, sometimes they will need your strength, too. You and your loved ones will fare better, if you have the courage to let yourselves grow stronger and closer because of what you are going through.

◆ The most important aspect of this is to not allow yourself to become isolated. You have family members, neighbors, friends, co-workers, other parishioners in your church, other supporters who care about some of the same local community issues. Keep the connective tissues between you and others nourished. Your circles of community can feed you and may, in fact, need what only you have to offer.

◆ Join a support group, if one is available. Consider starting one, if it is not established in your area. Even though you have some physical limitations, you can still make a contribution.

## LOCAL SUPPORT GROUPS

My own local support groups in southwest Michigan, are listed below as examples. If you find this book a valuable resource, I strongly encourage you to make copies of an insert card with your own local group information and enclose them in this book for possible use by other patients in your area.

◆ Kidney Club Support Group

Our mission: To provide a positive and encouraging source of education and support to all dialysis/transplant patients and their families.
Date:  The third Sunday of each month
Place:  Mr. Don's, 1275 E. Columbia
          Battle Creek, Michigan
Time: 1:30 p.m.
For more information: minerva_cc@yahoo.com

◆ LOTTS

Living Organ and Tissue Transplant Support Group

We are here to offer support to individuals who have already received transplants. To offer support and encouragement to individuals and their families who are waiting for an organ or tissue transplant. To Give support to donor families. To make the public aware of the need for organ and tissue donation.
Date: The second Tuesday of each month
Place: Community Room, Goldentree Apartments
          4795 E. Milham Rd.
          Kalamazoo, MI
Time:  7:00 p.m.
For further information contact:
P.O. Box 1424, Portage, MI. 49081-1424

## GLOSSARY

Please note that the following are non-technical defini-
tions to aid readers in general understanding. For a fuller
description of any listing, please consult your physician.

- **Antibiotic**: medicine to fight bacterial infections
- **Arterial/Venous**: access to blood supply
- **C.A.P.D.**: Continuos Ambulatory Peritoneal
  Dialysis.
- **C.C.A.P.D.**: Continuos Cycler Assisted Peritoneal
  Dialysis.
- **Catheter**: a flexible plastic tube used to bring
  fluids to or remove fluids from the body
- **Cycler**: a machine that assists with Peritoneal
  Dialysis, using a commercially prepared solution
  through the abdomen's semi-permeable membrane
  to rmove toxins and extra fluids from the blood.
- **Erythropoitin**: a medicine to increase blood pro-
  duction (Epo)
- **Fistula**: a surgically united segment of artery and
  vein
- **Hemodialysis**: the process of artificially circu-
  lating the blood outside the body through plastic
  tubes, filtering it in an artificial kidney and
  returning the clean blood back to the body.
- **Lupus**: an immune system disease that attacks the
  healthy tissues and organs
- **Pericardium**: lining around the heart

- **Pericarditis**: inflammation of the sac or fluid build-up around the lining surrounding the heart
- **Peritoneal**: lining inside the abdomen
- **Peritonitis**: infection inside the abdomen lining
- **Phosphorus**: essential element of blood; elevated levels can bind with calcium and cause calcification of soft tissues.

## RESOURCES THAT MIGHT BE USEFUL FOR ME